Paleo Diet

The Ultimate Beginner's Guide To Paleo Diet Plan - Proven Recipes to Lose Weight & Get Healthy with Modern Paleo Diet Meal Plan (Including 30+ Simple & Delicious Recipes)

By *Simone Jacobs*

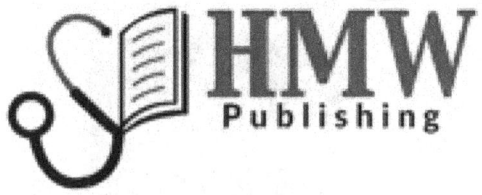

For more great books visit:

HMWPublishing.com

Get another book for Free

I want to thank you for purchasing this book and offer you another book (just as long and valuable as this book), "Health & Fitness Mistakes You Don't Know You're Making", completely free.

Visit the link below to signup and receive it:

www.hmwpublishing.com/gift

In this book, I will break down the most common health & fitness mistakes, you are probably committing right now, and I will reveal how you can easily get in the best shape of your life!

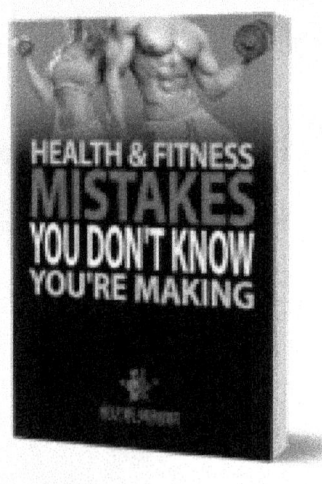

In addition to this valuable gift, you will also have an opportunity to get our new books for free, enter giveaways, and receive other valuable emails from me. Again, visit the link to sign up:

www.hmwpublishing.com/gift

TABLE OF CONTENTS

Introduction 5
Chapter 1: The Paleo diet 101 8
    Origin and Philosophy.. 8
Chapter 2: Benefits Of The Paleo Diet 11
Chapter 3: The Problem With The Current American Diet 17
    Problems with the Standard American Diet (SAD) 17
Chapter 4: Your Simple Paleo Food Guide ... 23
    Foods to avoid 23
    Foods to eat 26
Chapter 5: Making The Shift: Your 30-Day Challenge 29
Chapter 6: Awesome Paleo Recipes 33
    Breakfast 33
    Pumpkin Spiced Sweet Potato Spiral Waffle 33
    Baked Mashed Sweet Potatoes and Eggs 37
    Bacon and Avocado Omelets 39
    Menemen 41
    Breakfast Sausage Casserole 43
    Paleo Choco Waffles 45
    Baked Eggs and Bacon 47
    Mains 49
    Steak and Chimichurri Sauce 49
    Hamburger Steaks with Gravy Mushrooms 51

Honey Glazed Asian Salmon 54
Paleo Slow cooker Lasagna 56
Sweet Potato Pasta Topped With Buffalo Chicken Alfredo 60
Paleo Chow Mein 62
Spicy Beef with Bokchoy 65
Bacon-Basil Zucchini Pasta 67
Sweet Potato and Chicken Stew 69
Stuffed peppers with sausage 71
Peppered Shrimp 74
Deviled Crunchy Chicken 76
Avocado and Chicken Soup 78
Jambalaya Soup 80
Snacks 82
Bacon Choco Chip Cookies 82
Bacon Pumpkin Soup 84
Spicy Jicama Shoestring Fries 87
Quick Corn Salad 89
Easy Bake Kale Chips 91
Cucumber and Blueberry Smoothie 93
Apple Baked Chips 94
Grain-Free Brownie Bites 95
Quinoa Veggie Salad 96
Mint, Cucumber and Green Apple Smoothie 98
Kale and Pear Smoothie 99

Final Words 100

About the Co-Author 101

Introduction

I want to thank you and congratulate you for purchasing the *"Paleo Diet"* book. This book contains proven steps and strategies on how you can become healthy by following the wonderful world of the Paleo Diet. It has useful information on how you can follow and begin this eating lifestyle. There have been a lot of books and diets out in the market that continue to claim they can help you lose weight or become healthy. However, not all of them are effective, helpful or easy to follow. Choosing to be healthy and live a long life is never too late. You are the only one who holds that decision to change your life for the better and right you are heading to the right direction. If you are holding this book, congratulations! You are now part of the millions of people who want to experience the life-changing benefits of the Paleo Diet. In this book get to have an in-depth knowledge of this diet works. Learn its benefits, how to start the diet and make it work for you but above all, how to make it your lifestyle.

Always remember that in anything you do it is always

important to have determination and patience to be successful in any goal. So start right now and take action. Embark on a happy and nutritious Paleo journey! Thanks again for purchasing this book, I hope you enjoy it!

Also, before you get started, I recommend you **joining our email newsletter** to receive updates on any upcoming new book releases or promotions. You can sign-up for free, and as a bonus, you will receive a free gift. Our *"Health & Fitness Mistakes You Don't Know You're Making"* book! This book has been written to demystify, expose the top do's and don'ts and to finally equip you with the information you need to get in the best shape of your life. Due to the overwhelming amount of mis-information and lies told by magazines and self-proclaimed "gurus", it's becoming harder and harder to get reliable information to get in shape. As opposed to having to go through dozens of biased, unreliable and un-trustworthy sources to get your health & fitness information. Everything you need to help you has been broken down in this book for you to easily follow and to immediately get results to achieve your desired fitness goals in the shortest amount of time.

Once again, to join our free email newsletter and to receive a free copy of this valuable book, please visit the link and signup now: www.hmwpublishing.com/gift

CHAPTER 1: THE PALEO DIET 101

Paleo has evolved from just being a name. It is a lot more than only a mere "fad" diet as it has become a modern and healthy lifestyle. It is about nourishing the body with whole and natural foods, free from chemicals and other additives that are harmful to one's health. It is also known as the Paleolithic Diet or the "Caveman" Diet which is a way of eating wherein the focus is primarily on foods that our ancestors ate during the early times.

Origin and Philosophy

The history of the Paleo diet goes way back ago when man began to gather fruits, nuts and vegetables and hunt for animals in order to sustain themselves. There isn't a specific "founder" of the Paleo diet because man has been evolving and changing for millions and millions of years. However, this diet became popular during the 1970's by a gastroenterologist named Walter L. Voegtlin. He was one of the very first believers that this diet could improve the health and the well-being. He wrote the book "Stone Age Diet: Based on In-depth studies of Human Ecology and the Diet of Man" in 1975.

Early humans used to cultivate natural foods from the harvest. As man has evolved throughout the years, the food production has radically transformed as the population has grown. The introduction of chemicals in the production of foods, the drug injections to animals and pesticides applied to soil and foods are just a few examples of the industrialization era that we live today.

So if humans were not used to eating this kind of foods, then it means that this innovative system of food production is not necessarily healthy for the body. The question though is how come we have been eating these types of foods for so long, but nothing seemed to be wrong with us?

Unfortunately, that is not true! In fact, there have been studies, and sufficient evidence that is eating dairies, grains and a lot of processed foods lead to many diseases such as rheumatoid arthritis, type 2 diabetes, heart diseases, Crohn's diseases, multiple sclerosis, cancer and many other diseases.

And because of this alarming outcome, the Paleo Diet wants to teach you a new way of life – a healthy and happy life. To go back to the basics and practice clean eating – foods that are unprocessed, simple and natural. Paleo wants you to improve your eating habits thus helping you in the process to get rid of toxins in the body and minimize the risks of harmful diseases.

So look at it simply: our ancestors are eating whole and natural foods thus making them healthy, not overweight, full of energy and pretty much athletic. Today, you will notice that a lot of people have weight problems, are extremely stressed, some are suffering lack of sleep and have many other issues. The Paleo diet wants to change all of these things – this is an effort to improve the way people eat and adopt a healthy lifestyle.

Chapter 2: Benefits Of The Paleo Diet

The Paleo diet provides a lot of health benefits to many people. Upon observation with people who engaged in this diet, many confirmed that they had more energy within just a few weeks of following it. After a few more weeks, added benefits became evident like developing a leaner body and weight loss. These are the reasons why it is advisable to follow this diet thoroughly so that you can be able to see a big difference happen in your life. Read on and see the various benefits that the Paleo diet can bring you.

- **Weight loss**
  By design, this follows a low carbohydrate diet, and by removing processed foods in your eating habit, you will gain more fuel to help you lose weight.

- **More muscles in the body and less fat**
  Meat is one of the best sources of protein and proteins are suitable to be used for building new cells

that can help in making muscle mass. The more muscles you have, the leaner you will become, and the more chances of burning those unwanted fats can happen in the body and increase your metabolism.

- **Controlled blood sugar levels**

    If you are following the Paleo diet, it does not include any refined sugar, therefore, more natural for you to monitor your blood sugar levels especially if you are already in danger of being pre-diabetic. However, if you have diabetes, it is best to consult your doctor before you follow this diet.

- **Feeling full and nourished the whole day**

    One of the reasons why people eat a lot is because they get hungry immediately. The Paleo diet makes you feel full longer and lessens your tendency to eat more. Eating the right combination of meat and veggies will help you feel satisfied the whole day and not crave for foods that are bad for your health. With the addition of fruits, there is no need for you to pick up those sugary desserts that would only make you feel more sluggish and irritable.

- **Prevention of diseases**

    Since the primary focus of the Paleo diet is eating natural and whole foods, you automatically eliminate processed foods from your system and instead you eat more foods that are rich in phytonutrients and antioxidants that help in preventing a lot of diseases such as cancer or heart diseases.

- **No calorie count needed**

    Unlike other diets that require strict compliance when it comes to eating food, the Paleo diet is fun, easy and straightforward to follow. There are no limitations on the amount of food you are allowed to eat. As long as you eat as our ancestors ate before, there is no need for you to keep on counting those calories.

- **Provides more energy**

    The combination of the approved Paleo foods will provide a balanced meal that is rich in protein, carbohydrates, vitamins, and minerals especially if they are eaten consistently and in the right manner. Unlike other diets that are restrictive, the Paleo diet allows you to eat whenever you are hungry, eliminating the risk of making you feel weak and low on energy.

- **Better sleep condition and controls mood changes**

    By avoiding processed food, you avoid ingesting additives and chemicals, thus helping your brain release serotonin, a chemical secreted by the body that acts as a neurotransmitter, helping you relax and fall asleep naturally. Aside from that, you will also have better mood balance leading to a happier disposition of life.

- **Provides Detoxifying Effects for the body**

    Stopping the intake of foods that are rich in chemicals, additives like refined sugar, gluten, trans-fats and others will allow your body to take a rest and heal itself naturally. The more you eat fruits and veggies, the more antioxidants are being produced, helping you to eliminate wastes and toxins that are already present in the body. Think of it as a natural detoxifier. You don't need to experience starvation or engage in extreme measures like fasting to detoxify.

- **Healthier gut**

    Sugar, processed junk and unhealthy fats can cause inflammation in your intestines. When you eat too much-processed foods coupled with a lot of stress, you will have a "leaky gut syndrome" where the walls of your intestine are damaged and the things that do not leave inside your gut leaks out. Engaging in the Paleo diet will help to avoid having such problems as you eat less processed foods and healthier foods.

These are just some of the significant benefits the Paleo diet can bring you. With the right attitude and mindset, you will be able to achieve this goal and help you live a healthy and longer life.

Chapter 3: The Problem With The Current American Diet

In today's society, people want convenience and speed because of their busy lifestyle. Hence the majority of the population engage in unhealthy habits which include food intake. They tend to eat and eat relentlessly not knowing that sometimes the food they eat is not suitable for their health which leads to an unhealthy way of life.

Problems with the Standard American Diet (SAD)

What is the Standard American Diet?

If you are given a list of food that you encounter every day when eating out, you will find that they are very high in fat, low in fiber, very high in calories and high in salt content. These are the perfect formula present for the SAD. It consists of many things that your body mostly "do not necessarily need." The worst thing about this is that it is no longer the "standard diet" in America alone, they are also becoming a problem worldwide. Many industrialized countries are now engaged in this type of eating habits because foods that are processed can easily be attained and are available almost everywhere.

Studies have shown that almost 63% of calories that American people consume come from processed or refined foods like potato chips, soft drinks, french fries and more. Only a mere 6% comes from fruits and vegetables and other healthy grains – something that people should get worried about.

Hence these are the reasons why people are becoming sick and more people are acquiring illnesses that sometimes lead to early death. Take a look at the other effects SAD can bring to an individual. Also, take note that these are also reasons why people are becoming sluggish and sickly as well:

Promotes bad eating habits

It is so difficult to balance career and family life, and that is the truth! Hence, people settle for choosing fast food or prepared meals to satisfy their hunger. Many people have no choice, and some don't have the time to develop their food or choose healthier food products. Most of the time they will just settle for a slice of pizza, hamburgers, french fries, and sodas – and this will not make people healthy.

Processed foods and packed foods have become so prevalent because of its convenience and quicker food preparation, which these are the reasons why people just keep on consuming. For them, it is the perfect alternative to provide quick meals for themselves and their family as well.

Frequent consumption of carbonated and sugary drinks has also been prevalent in today's society. Aside from having too much sugar and calories, it also contributes to fast body dehydration hence making people feel tired most of the time.

Opting to too much technology

While technology brought forth so many advantages, it also has its disadvantages. Modern technology teaches people to become lazy and immobile. Instead, a simple flick of a button, people don't need to stand up anymore to turn on appliances.

What is more, with the prominence of the internet, there is no need for people to get out, socialize or even pay their bills. The internet conveniently provides everything for people – from entertainment, shopping, education – why the need to go out anyway?

Gaming consoles are baby sitters for children. Most parents only allow their kids to stay in front of their computers or gaming consoles for hours while they are busy doing their work. There are no more socialization and movement!

People have become addicted to technology that they tend to forget the simpler things in life. They have grown so engrossed in their tablets, smartphones or laptops not knowing that constant exposure to these devices may have effects on their health in the long run. Sleep has been compromised hence they always feel so sluggish or tired in the morning.

Lack of movement

It's quite simple to understand that when a person lacks movement or do not move at all, they become sluggish and gain more weight. This is also in connection with taking focus on too much technology. With hours and hours in front of your computer or gaming console, do you think that you are doing such a significant job burning calories or becoming active? I guess you already knew the answer.

Being inactive is one of the culprits of why people become fat and accumulate many diseases. Instead of giving your body time to burn calories or make it lean and fit, it stays dormant hence the reason why people also feels tired and sluggish most of the time.

Lack of Sleep

Because the SAD diet is rich in sugar, people are having difficulty creating a good night sleep. Sugar makes people hyperactive hence instead of calming the nerves; it keeps the senses awake at all times. Getting a right amount of zzz's is very important as this will help in the development of cells and muscles in the body. It also improves the mood and state of mind of an individual come the next day. Eating healthy foods helps in calming the nerves and triggers sleep-inducing hormones that will allow people to have a good night's rest.

It is essential that every individual has a good solid 8-9 hour of sleep. Experts say that this is the time that every cell in the body is developing, muscles are rebuilding itself and help in replenishing used up energy after a day's tough work.

Changing times means it is also about time for you to turn and take charge of yourself. The Paleo diet is here to help you as long as you want to. In the next chapter, you will learn more about what foods to eat when you engage in this healthy diet.

Chapter 4: Your Simple Paleo Food Guide

This chapter will provide you an idea of what food that the diet allows. Here are the basics:

DO EAT: veggies, fish, eggs, meat, fruits, herb, spices, nuts, seeds, healthy oils, and fats

DON'T EAT: sugar, processed foods, soft drinks, most dairy products, grains, legumes, vegetable oils, margarine, artificial sweeteners, and trans-fats

Foods to avoid

- *Dairy*

   Dairy food including its by-products should be eliminated. However, there are some versions of the diet that allow full-fat dairies like cheese and butter.

- *Cereal grains*

Avoid eating foods that have grains in them. This includes corn, pancakes, cereals, oatmeal, kinds of pasta, bread, barley and more.

- *Legumes this include peanuts*

  As mentioned, peanuts are not allowed because, in reality, they are legumes. Legumes are rich in carbohydrates and packed with gluten that is bad for the health. So as much as possible, avoid these types of foods especially peanuts.

- *Refined sugar or artificial sweeteners*

  By definition itself, "artificial," meaning synthetic or modified. This includes sucralose, cyclamates, aspartame, saccharin, acesulfame potassium. Therefore, if you would like to add sweetness to your dish, use natural sweeteners.

- *Processed foods, junk foods, and candies*

  Just like artificial sweeteners, processed foods are not Paleo. These foods are rich in additives and artificial flavorings that are bad for the health. Sugar present in today's foods is addictive, making you want to eat more. Stay away from these types of foods.

- *Refined vegetable oils, trans-fats*

   Avoid using processed oils in your cooking. Make sure to find other alternative healthy oils like olive oil or coconut oil.

- *Starchy veggies*

   This includes your favorite potatoes and sweet potatoes. Avoid them because they are rich and loaded with starch.

- *Too much salty food*

   Yes, it's hard to eat food that tastes bland, but too much salt is bad for your health. This can lead to many adverse effects such as hypertension and high cholesterol levels. Try adding herbs to your dish to make it tastier instead of adding too much salt.

- *Sodas and fruit juices*

    These beverages are rich in sugar and are not Paleo. Remove them from your diet.

- *Energy drinks & alcoholic drinks*

Foods to eat

- *Grass-fed or "organic" meats*

    Almost all of the meats are included in the Paleo diet but meat-derived foods like hot dogs, Spam or sausages are a no-no.

- *Fish and seafood*

    All types of fish can definitely be eaten especially if they are cooked in a simple way like steamed or broiled.

- *Fresh fruits and veggies*

    Almost all kinds of vegetables are included in this

diet like broccoli, peppers, onions, carrots, kale etc.

Fruits on the other hand are also included but you should take note that they contain sugar. Unlike veggies, try to look out for fruits that have high fructose content especially if you are on a diet. Eat them in moderation.

- *Nuts and Seeds*

    All nuts are indeed Paleo in nature and this is the best alternative to chips or fries and can be eaten as snacks. However, you need to be careful in eating cashew nuts for they are rich in fat. So in case you are trying to lose weight, eat in moderation or might as well avoid it.

- *Eggs*

    They are another good source of protein and energy for the body. You can either eat chicken, goose or duck eggs but make sure that they are free-range or pastured.

- *Healthy oils (like walnut, olive, flaxseed, avocado, macadamia, coconut)*
  Natural fats and oils are the best types of oils that you can use for cooking. They are also good sources of energy aside from being healthy.

In the past years, the community of Paleo diet have already evolved, and there are now several versions or additions to the diet. Some already include bacon as long as it came from grass-fed pigs. They also added butter and some non-gluten grains like rice.

There are also some indulgences that are included in drinking quality red wine and dark chocolate. Make sure that your body is replenished well by drinking plenty of water. Most people include tea and coffee in the diet as they are both rich in antioxidants.

Chapter 5: Making The Shift: Your 30-Day Challenge

The Paleo Diet is said to be the diet of cavemen, where they only eat healthy food, such as fish, eggs, and vegetables. You focus on eating food that will give you enough protein to support healthy muscles and provide you with optimal immune function. However, if you are still new to the Paleo Diet and even don't know if this is the one for you below are some tips and tricks which can help you determine if it is the diet for you. By following this simple guide, you can determine how to make Paleo Diet work for you.

Determine your real motivation for taking this diet. While people make the Paleo Diet lose weight, there are also other benefits. By researching, you determine your real motivation for choosing this diet. Look at your health situation and see what weighs the most. Do you have a big tummy and want to lessen the fats? Or, do you just want to be healthy every day, so you can have more energy to do things? There are many reasons why people take the Paleo

Diet. By determining your motivation, you can create a plan. And if you want to achieve your goal, be strict in following your program for at least a one month.

Clean your kitchen. When you have decided to take the Paleo Diet, you should be aware that there is food that you cannot eat. The moment you start the diet, clean out your kitchen. And clean, we mean removing all the "no" food, such as dairy, cheese, packaged and processed, oils. Throw them or give them away to someone else, but remove it from your household. By doing this, you avoid the temptation that can ruin your diet because basically, the food is not there.

However, if you want to take things slow, you can start removing the dairy first, then the grains in the next week, and then the processed food in the third week---and so forth. It takes time, but at least you can restock your kitchen with healthy and beneficial food that will make your better.

Learn how to cook on your own. Trying the Paleo Diet means you don't have to eat out anymore every day. This is because the diet consists of whole, fresh food that can be used to create meals at home. You can control the ingredients because you follow guidelines and you look at what you cook. Thanks to the diet, you can experiment with new dishes using the ingredients allowed by the Paleo diet. When you prepare, you can cook healthier meals and even try other ingredients in your cooking. About that, research on Paleo recipes for inspiration, so your meals are both flavorful and healthy.

Change your plate. Most of the time, our plates consist of grains, some vegetables, and meat. Scrap that and concentrate on having a balanced plate. Fill it with a palm-sized portion of protein, a few fats, and the rest are veggies, veggies, and veggies. Change your plate with different vegetables because you can never go wrong with it. As much as possible, avoid the grains because that is not part of the diet. If you can, put some fruits in between meals as well. For sure, you will feel great and healthy afterward.

Stick with the program for at least 30 days: most people have difficulty in switching diets, and that's true. There will be moments that your body will crave for the foods that you eliminate and you might feel sluggish or terrible the first few weeks. That's why it is essential to follow the diet for at least 30 days to allow your body to cope up with the changes. Remember that you want to succeed with your goal – whether losing weight or becoming healthy.

Lastly, even if you are on a diet, you can still eat out in restaurants---but with caution. Sometimes, it is okay to eat out with your friends in a restaurant. However, once you are aware of the ingredients you need in the Paleo Diet, you can use that skill in ordering food. According to Stephenson, "you can look at the menu ahead of time and pick one or two options that you can Paleo-size." Most of the time, it involves fish and vegetables. Also, don't hesitate to ask how the food is prepared and on making changes.

These are just some of the tips that you can follow when you plan to start the Paleo Diet. You don't have to hurry in trying it out because you can do it slowly. By taking things step-by-step, you will be on the road to a healthier you.

Chapter 6: Awesome Paleo Recipes

Here are some of the great recipes that you can try out yourself

Breakfast

Pumpkin Spiced Sweet Potato Spiral Waffle

Ingredients

- 1 piece sweet potato (medium sized spiralized in Blade C)
- 1 teaspoon of pumpkin spice
- 1 section beaten medium egg
- Cooking spray
- 1 tablespoon of maple syrup (you can add depending on your taste)

Directions

1. Heat the waffle iron.

2. Coat a large skillet with cooking spray and place it on a burner over medium heat.

3. Cook the sweet potato spirals in the skillet, carefully turning them regularly. Cook for about 10 minutes or until the spirals have softened completely.

4. Place them in a bowl and sprinkle it with pumpkin spice. Combine them until coated evenly. Then add the beaten egg and gently mix.

5. Check if waffle iron is hot. Once heated up, spray it with the cooking spray and put in the sweet potato spiral mix. Make sure to fit the sweet potato spiral mix in the waffle iron and cook them according to its setting.

6. Drizzle with maple syrup, serve and enjoy!

Paleo Muffins

Ingredients

- 6 eggs
- 6 tablespoons of melted coconut oil
- 1 teaspoon of vanilla extract
- ¼ teaspoon of sea salt
- 1 teaspoon of baking powder
- ½ cup of coconut flour
- ½ cup of frozen fruits (you can use any of your favorite fruits; this recipe used raspberries)

Directions

1. Preheat your oven to 400 degrees.
2. Combine all of the ingredients except the frozen fruits. Mix them well.
3. Fold in the frozen fruit. Pour the batter into muffin cups and bake for about 15 minutes. You can tell if

the muffins are thoroughly cooked if you place a toothpick in the middle and when it comes out, it is clean.

4. Cool before serving. Enjoy!

Baked Mashed Sweet Potatoes and Eggs

Ingredients

- 1 medium-sized sweet potato
- 1 small sized onion
- 1 tablespoon of EVOO (extra virgin olive oil)
- 2 medium-sized beets (boiled)
- 4 eggs
- 1 tablespoon of Mrs. Dash original blend seasoning

Directions

1. Preheat your oven to 350 degrees.
2. Grate sweet potatoes using your grater or if you have a food processor that has the grating feature, use it. It is faster and more comfortable. Finely chop the onions.
3. Using your frying pan, heat olive oil on high flame. Add onion, sweet potatoes, and Mrs. Dash seasoning. Mix well and cook until it becomes soft and brown.

4. Slice the beets to create the crust. Using a 9x9 baking pan, grease and place the sweet potato hash on top. Create holes to provide space for your eggs.

5. Crack the eggs on the hash and bake this for about 15-20 minutes. Check if the desired consistency of the egg is okay with you. Once done, take out of the oven and serve. Enjoy!

Bacon and Avocado Omelets

Ingredients

- 1 piece of avocado (pitted and flesh scooped)
- 2 tablespoons of red onion (minced)
- 4 bacon slices
- A dash of hot sauce
- 4 eggs
- 1 tablespoon of cilantro (minced)

Directions

1. Cook the bacon until it becomes crisp.
2. Meanwhile, mash the avocado flesh until smooth but not too much. A little texture is okay.
3. Add cilantro and onion. Once bacon is crisp, drain on a paper towel and crumble. Add the avocado mixture.

4. Whisk your eggs and cook in the pan. Make an omelet and place half of the avocado mixture in the middle. Repeat the same in the other omelet.

5. Transfer to plate and add hot sauce if you want. Serve and enjoy!

Menemen

Ingredients

- 1 medium sized tomato (diced)
- 1 tablespoon of olive oil
- ¼ red onion (diced)
- ½ cup of diced bell pepper (green)
- 1 clove of crushed garlic
- ¼ teaspoon of black pepper
- ¼ teaspoon of cumin (ground)
- ¼ teaspoon of salt
- ¼ teaspoon of turmeric
- ¼ teaspoon of red pepper flakes
- 3 eggs
- 1 tablespoon of parsley (minced)

Directions

1. Using a big pan, heat oil and saute tomato, onion and bell pepper. Add the crushed garlic plus the cumin, pepper flakes, turmeric and black pepper as well. Stir and cook until veggies are cooked.

2. Meanwhile, crack the eggs and whisk. Add in the pan and gently stir until eggs are fully incorporated. It would then have a creamy consistency.

3. Ladle on a bowl, top with parsley, serve hot and enjoy!

Breakfast Sausage Casserole

Ingredients

- 1 lb of Italian sausage (remove the casings)
- 2 pieces of diced sweet potatoes
- 8 eggs
- 1 diced medium onion
- 1 diced bell pepper
- 1/3 cup of coconut milk or almond milk
- 3 cloves of minced garlic
- 2 thinly sliced green onions
- Pepper and salt for tasting
- Coconut oil, butter or ghee for cooking

Directions

1. Preheat your oven to 375 degrees F.

2. Heat oil in a pan over medium to high heat then add sausages. Crumble it while you are cooking. Once cooked, transfer in a large sized bowl. Set aside.

3. Add garlic, bell pepper and onion in the same pan. Cook for about 4-5 minutes on medium heat. Transfer them to the bowl with the sausages and mix in the sweet potatoes as well. Mix to combine well.

4. Pour the mixture into a baking dish.

5. In a separate bowl, whisk eggs, pepper, salt and almond milk. Pour it over the sweet potato and sausage mix.

6. Bake for about 20 minutes. Top with green onions. Serve hot and enjoy!

Paleo Choco Waffles

Ingredients

For the pancake batter

- 4 eggs
- 4 tablespoons of coconut flour
- 1 cup of applesauce
- 1 cup of almond flour
- ¼ teaspoon of sea salt
- ½ teaspoon of vanilla
- ½ teaspoon of baking soda
- ¼ cup of dark choco chips
- 4 tablespoons of cocoa powder

For the chocolate sauce:

- 2 tablespoons of coconut oil
- ¼ cup of dark choco chips

Directions

1. Prepare the waffle batter by mixing all of the ingredients in a bowl. Blend until combined well. Turn on your waffle iron to high then pour enough mixture and cook for about 4 to 5 minutes. Repeat the whole procedure.

2. Meanwhile, place the choco chips and coconut oil using a small saucepan over low heat. Melt chocolate and whisk to combine fully.

3. Pour choco syrup over cooked waffles. Serve and enjoy!

Baked Eggs and Bacon

Ingredients

- 2 tablespoons of butter //
- 4 large sized eggs
- 1 cup of cheddar cheese (grated)
- 1 cup of heavy cream (heated until warm)
- 8 slices of bacon (cooked and crumbled)
- Pepper and salt for tasting

Directions

1. Preheat your oven to 350 degrees. Spread some butter to 4 small ceramic ramekins or small glasses.
2. Break the egg on each of the ramekin.
3. Cover the eggs with ¼ cup of the heated cream and ¼ cup cheese. Season it with pepper and salt.
4. Put the ramekins in a pan and fill it with water, just enough to become half on the sides of the ramekins.

Bake for about 15 minutes or until cheese melts thoroughly and the whites of the eggs are done.

5. Crumble some slices of bacon on top of each egg. Serve hot and enjoy!

Mains

Steak and Chimichurri Sauce

Ingredients

- A pound of beef flap steak (choose the sirloin part)
- ½ cup of parsley (flat leaf)
- 1 cup of arugula
- ½ teaspoon of red pepper flakes
- 2 ½ tablespoons of vinegar (white wine)
- 2 cloves of garlic
- ¼ cup of olive oil
- ¼ teaspoon of salt
- ¼ teaspoon of pepper

Directions

1. Heat your grill to medium to high heat. Season your steak with pepper and salt.

2. Meanwhile using your food processor, combine other ingredients to make the sauce. Set aside.

3. Grill your steak around 2 to 3 minutes on each side until charred. Transfer to plate and let rest for about 5 minutes.

4. Once the steak is rested, carve steak and serve with the sauce. Enjoy!

Hamburger Steaks with Gravy Mushrooms

Ingredients

- 1 lb of ground beef
- 3 tablespoons of fresh parsley (chopped and add more for garnishing)
- 3 tablespoons of minced garlic
- 1 tablespoon of powdered onion
- 1 tablespoon of powdered garlic
- ½ teaspoon of sea salt
- ½ teaspoon of freshly cracked peppers
- 2 tablespoons of apple cider vinegar
- 1 cup of diced onions
- 8 ounces of packed fresh mushrooms (sliced)
- 1 cup of beef stock

- 1 can of coconut milk

- 2 tablespoons of arrowroot powder

- 2 tablespoons of bacon fat (or you can use other cooking fat)

- 2 tablespoons of grass-fed butter (to make it more paleo instead of primal, you can use coconut oil)

Directions

1. Using a large sized mixing bowl, combine ground beef, garlic and all of the dry seasoning ingredients. Mix well and form them to patties.

2. In a separate saucepan, melt bacon fat and start searing the beef patties on both sides, 2 minutes each side. Set aside.

3. Reduce heat and melt butter. Add mushrooms and onions constantly stirring for about 5-9 minutes until mushrooms are tender. Pour beef stock, apple cider vinegar and coconut milk.

4. Meanwhile, dissolve the arrowroot powder with water and stir well. Mix with the gravy mixture and continue to simmer on low heat for about 20 minutes.

5. Add the beef patties in the gravy and simmer again for another 20 minutes until the gravy seeps its flavor with the patties.

6. Transfer to plate and add gravy on top.

7. Garnish with chopped parsley. Serve and enjoy!

Honey Glazed Asian Salmon

Ingredients

- 2 tablespoons of honey
- 2 tablespoons of coconut aminos
- 1 teaspoon of apple cider vinegar
- ½ inched size grated fresh ginger
- ½ teaspoon of lime juice
- 2 pieces of (6 ounces) salmon fillets
- 1 tablespoon of coconut oil
- 1 tablespoon of chopped cilantro
- Sesame seed for garnishing

Directions

1. Preheat your oven to 400 degrees.
2. Using a small-sized bowl, combine honey, vinegar, coconut aminos, lime juice and ginger. Set them aside. This is the honey glaze mixture.

3. Melt coconut oil using an safe oven pan. Cook salmon with skin facing side up. Sear for about 3-4 minutes until it becomes brown.

4. Flip and drizzle using half of honey glaze mixture. Pop the skillet inside the oven and bake for about 5-6 minutes or until salmon is cooked according to your preference.

5. Remove from the oven and transfer to a serving plate.

6. Drizzle remaining honey glaze on top.

7. Sprinkle with sesame seeds and cilantro.

8. Serve and enjoy!

Paleo Slow cooker Lasagna

Ingredients

For the Marinara Sauce

- ¼ cup of olive oil
- 1 small sized onion (diced)
- 1 teaspoon of salt
- 7 cups of tomatoes (about 10 tomatoes; diced)
- ½ teaspoon of raw honey

For the Meat Filling

- 1 tablespoon of olive oil
- ½ small sized onion (diced)
- 1 pound of ground turkey
- ½ teaspoon of pepper
- 18 pieces of basil leaves (chopped)

For the cheese sauce

- ½ teaspoon of olive oil

- ¼ small sized onion (chopped)

- ½ summer squash (chopped)

- ½ teaspoon of garlic (minced)

- ¼ teaspoon of salt

- ½ cup of coconut milk

- 1 egg

- 4 medium-sized zucchini (sliced thinly)

Directions

1. Using a large sized saucepan, heat olive oil over medium-high heat. Sauté the onions and add salt for about 2 minutes. Add garlic and sauté again for another 30 seconds. Once garlic turned fragrant, add honey and tomatoes and reduce heat. Let cook for around 20 minutes or until the sauce thickens. Season to taste. Adjust according to your preference.

2. To prepare the meat filling, in another pan, heat olive oil over medium-high heat. Cook ground turkey for about 2 minutes. Add salt, onion, and pepper. Continue to cook until turkey is cooked thoroughly. Remove from heat and add basil leaves. Set aside.

3. To prepare the cheese sauce, get a small-sized saucepan. Heat olive oil over medium-high heat. Sauté summer squash, onions, garlic and salt for around 3-4 minutes until onions become translucent. Make sure that this would not turn brown. Add ¼ cup of coconut milk and bring to boil. Simmer for about 2 minutes or until half of liquid becomes fully absorbed.

4. Using a blender, pour the mixture and blend well adding the ¼ cup of coconut milk. Blend well until it turned very smooth. Add egg and mix again. Make sure that it becomes well blended.

5. To assemble the lasagna, grease the insides of a slow cooker. Cover the bottom with ¾ cups of marinara sauce and spread it evenly.

6. Arrange around 5 zucchini "slices/noodles" on top of the marinara sauce. Spoon a layer of "cheese sauce" on top of the zucchini and put a generous amount of the turkey filling. Spoon again around ½-3/4 cups of marina sauce over the turkey filling. Spread it evenly. Repeat the same process until the first portion will end with the marinara sauce.

7. Cover and cook it for about 1 ½ hours over high heat. Remove lid and ladle excess liquid on the surface. Zucchini will also produce a few amount of fluid. Place the excess liquid in a shallow pan.

8. Bring to boil the excess liquid. Simmer it around 5-7 minutes until the sauce becomes thick and creamy.

9. Pour the reduced sauce on top of the lasagna inside the slow cooker. Place lasagna on a plate. Serve hot and enjoy!

Sweet Potato Pasta Topped With Buffalo Chicken Alfredo

Ingredients:

- 1 pound of chicken (poached or broiled)
- 3 pieces of spiralized sweet potato
- 3 tablespoons of oil (for cooking the sweet potato spirals)
- 1 cup of heavy coconut cream or heavy cream (from the can)
- 1 tablespoon of butter
- 4 teaspoon of starch (either Arrowroot, Potato Starch or Tapioca)
- 2 tablespoons of hot sauce
- ¼ teaspoon of powdered garlic
- ¼ to ½ teaspoon of powdered chili (optional)
- Salt and pepper to taste

Directions

1. Combine cream, butter, hot sauce, starch, salt, pepper, powdered garlic and powdered chili in a saucepan. Whisk the ingredients until sauce thickens then set aside.

2. Cook the chicken in a skillet or poach them then set aside.

3. Cook the sweet potato spirals over medium-high heat in a medium saucepan. Occasionally, check them until they are cooked thoroughly.

4. Once done, combine the cooked sweet potato spirals, chicken, and the sauce. Mix and toss lightly.

5. Serve hot and enjoy!

Paleo Chow Mein

Ingredients:

- ½ pound of chicken, cut into 1-in. strips
- ½ tablespoons of ghee
- 1 tablespoons of coconut aminos
- 1 tablespoons of rice vinegar
- ½ green cabbage, cored and thinly sliced
- 1 large carrot, shredded
- 1 small broccoli, stemmed and cut into bite-size pieces
- 2 zucchinis, spiraled

For the sauce:

- 3 tablespoons of coconut aminos
- 2 tablespoons of rice vinegar
- 1 teaspoon of sesame oil

- 1 tablespoon of fish sauce

- 2-inch ginger, fresh, minced

- 2 cloves of garlic, minced

- 1 teaspoon of honey

- ¼ teaspoon of sriracha

Directions

1. In a large wok over medium-high heat, melt the ghee. Add the chicken, 1 tablespoon of coconut aminos, and 1 tablespoon of rice vinegar. Stir all together and cook for 5-7 minutes.

2. In another separate bowl, whisk together all the sauce ingredients. Add the cabbage, carrot, and broccoli into the sauce and toss until well covered.

3. Mix all these in the large wok and stir. Cook for another 10-15 minutes or until the cabbage is wilted by occasional stirring, covered.

4. Add the zucchini noodles and allow to cook for another 7-10 minutes.

5. Serve and enjoy!

Spicy Beef with Bokchoy

Ingredients

- 12 heads of baby bok choy (cut it lengthwise)
- 1 piece of onion (sliced thinly)
- 2 lbs of beef sirloin (sliced thinly to strips)
- 2 tablespoons of fish sauce
- 2 cloves of minced garlic
- 3 teaspoons of coconut oil
- 1 piece of small minced ginger
- 5 pieces of red chiles (dried; halved; if desired)
- Pepper and salt for tasting

Directions

1. Season beef with pepper and salt. Heat coconut oil using a big pan over high heat.

2. Add garlic, chiles if you will use and ginger. Stir fry for about a minute until they become aromatic. Add

beef then cook for another 2-3 more minutes. Transfer to bowl.

3. Using another skillet, saute onions for about 2 minutes then add bok choy. Cook for another 3-4 minutes until it becomes soft.

4. Return back the beef to the skillet then add fish sauce. Stir and combine well. Serve hot and enjoy!

Bacon-Basil Zucchini Pasta

Ingredients

- 4 large zucchinis, spiraled
- 2 teaspoons of salt
- 1/3 cup of bacon grease
- ¼ cup of fresh basil, chopped
- 2 cloves of garlic, crushed
- ½ cup of walnuts, chopped

Directions

1. Season the zucchini with salt and let it sit into a sieve for at least 20 minutes to drain out the water. Rinse and then place it into a paper towel to squeeze and remove the excess moisture.

2. In a frying pan over medium-high heat, put in the bacon grease. Saute the garlic and zucchini by frequent stirring for about 4-5 minutes or until cooked 'al Dante.'

3. Toss in the basil and walnuts and allow to cook for another 2 minutes with occasional stirring.

4. Serve and enjoy!

Sweet Potato and Chicken Stew

Ingredients

- 6 pieces of chicken thigh (bone-in; remove the skin and trim the fat)
- 2 pounds of sweet potatoes (cut to spears and peeled)
- ½ pound of button mushrooms (use the white type; sliced thinly)
- 6 large-sized shallots (cut to half and peeled)
- 4 cloves of peeled garlic
- 1 cup of white wine (dry)
- 2 teaspoons of fresh rosemary (chopped; you can also use ½ teaspoon of crushed dried rosemary)
- 1 teaspoon of salt
- ½ teaspoon of fresh ground pepper
- 1 ½ tablespoons of vinegar (white wine)

Directions

1. Place sweet potatoes, chicken, shallots, garlic, shallots, mushrooms, pepper, salt, rosemary and wine in the slow cooker and cover.

2. Cook around 5 hours on low or until the sweet potatoes become tender. Once done, you can choose to remove the bones before serving.

3. Ladle into serving bowls. Serve hot and enjoy!

Stuffed peppers with sausage

Ingredients

- 1 lb. of Italian hot sausage (ground)
- 5 pieces of different bell peppers (yellow, red, green)
- ½ head of cauliflower (chopped and grated into rice-like consistency)
- 1 small (8 oz.) canned tomato paste
- 1 small sized white onion (diced)
- ½ head garlic (minced)
- 1 fresh basil (minced or you can use 2 teaspoons of dried basil)
- 2 teaspoon of oregano (dried)
- 2 teaspoon of thyme (dried)

Directions

1. To prepare the peppers: cut the top off and scrape out the seeds. Do not throw the tops. You will still be using it later.

2. Finely chop half of the head of the cauliflower turning it into a rice consistency. Place it in a large sized mixing bowl.

3. Add basil, herbs, garlic, and onions and mix it lightly.

4. Meanwhile, lightly brown sausages over high heat on a pan. You can choose to skip this step because the sausage will be cooked when added to the slow cooker. However, searing the sausages will bring out more flavors and liven up the dish.

5. Once done searing, add the sausages on the bowl of cauliflower together with the canned tomato paste and mix well. Make sure to mix this by hand.

6. When you are already done mixing, place mixture inside the peppers. Put in as much as possible to make it compact but be careful not to break the whole

peppers. Include pepper tops so that they will also be cooked.

7. Place them in a slow cooker and cook for about 6 hours.

8. Once cooked, transfer to a plate. Serve hot and enjoy!

Peppered Shrimp

Ingredients

- 3 tablespoons of coconut oil
- 1 ½ lb of shrimp (peeled with tails on)
- 4 cloves of minced garlic
- 1 tablespoon of coconut aminos
- 1 teaspoon of black pepper
- 1 tablespoon of fish sauce
- ¼ cup of fresh cilantro (chopped)

Directions

1. Place a big and heavy skillet over low heat. Melt the coconut oil and saute minced garlic. Saute for about 2-3 minutes until fragrant.

2. Add in shrimp and cook for about 4-5 minutes or until it becomes pink. Add coconut aminos, pepper and fish sauce. Cook for another minute or two.

Transfer shrimp to plate once done together with the liquid. Top with cilantro. Serve and enjoy!

Deviled Crunchy Chicken

Ingredients

- 4 piece of chicken legs (thigh and leg quarters)
- 1 teaspoon of curry powder
- 1 teaspoon of dry mustard
- ½ cup of almond meal
- 4 tablespoons of olive oil
- 1 teaspoon of cayenne powder

Directions

1. Preheat your oven to 350 degrees F.
2. Separate legs from thighs then rub each of the pieces with a small amount of olive oil.
3. Meanwhile combine almond meal, cayenne, curry powder and dry mustard. Combine it well.
4. Roll the chicken parts on the almond meal mixture then arrange them over a sheet pan.

5. Roast for about an hour or more or until the juices are clear when you pierce it through the bone. Make sure that the coating turned crunchy as well.

6. Serve and enjoy!

Avocado and Chicken Soup

Ingredients

- 1 teaspoon of Sriracha (for tasting)
- 1 lb of chicken breast (boneless and skinless)
- 6 cups of chicken broth
- 4 scallions (slice, separate the green and white part)
- 1 diced avocado
- 1 clove of crushed garlic
- Pepper and salt for tasting

Directions

1. Pour your broth in a large and heavy pan. Heat on medium to high heat. Add Sriracha and let the broth simmer.

2. Add chicken and white part of scallions. Let simmer then add crushed garlic. Continue to simmer for about 20 minutes. Add pepper and salt.

3. Once done, ladle into serving bowls. Top with sliced avocado and green scallions. Serve and enjoy!

Jambalaya Soup

Ingredients

- 5 cups of chicken stock
- 4 pieces of chopped bell peppers (any color will do)
- 1 large sized chopped onion
- 1 large canned organic tomatoes (diced)
- 2 cloves of diced garlic
- 2 pieces of bay leaf
- 1 pound of large-sized shrimp (peeled and de-veined)
- 4 ounces of diced chicken
- 1 package of Andouille sausage (spicy)
- ½ to 1 head of cauliflower
- 2 cups of okra (if desired)
- 3 tablespoons of Cajun seasoning
- ¼ cup of hot sauce

Directions

1. Place the chicken, garlic, chopped bell peppers, onion, Cajun seasoning, hot sauce, and bay leaf in the slow cooker. Add chicken stock and cover. Cook for 6 hours on low.

2. 30 minutes before the soup base is done, add sausage. Meanwhile, pulse the cauliflower using a food processor to make cauliflower rice. Add it on the jambalaya on the last 20 minutes including the shrimp.

3. Once done, ladle on serving bowls. Serve hot and enjoy!

Snacks

Bacon Choco Chip Cookies

Ingredients

- 2 cups of almond flour
- ¼ teaspoon of salt
- ¼ teaspoon of baking soda
- 6 tablespoons of melted coconut oil
- 4 tablespoons of honey
- 2 teaspoon of vanilla extract
- 2 tablespoons of coconut milk
- 4-6 tablespoons of bacon (crumbled and cooked)
- ½ cup of chocolate chips

Directions

1. Preheat your oven to 350 degrees.

2. Meanwhile using a parchment paper, line the cookie tray.

3. Combine almond flour, salt, and baking soda. Mix them well using a fork.

4. In a separate bowl, combine all of the wet ingredients. Make sure that the coconut oil is melted.

5. Mix the dry and wet ingredients and fold in the bacon crumbs gently. Do not over stir. Fold in well enough to be combined thoroughly. This is now your cookie mixture.

6. Form small balls using your hands and place them on the cookie sheet. Bake for about 8-10 minutes or until it becomes brown on top. Serve hot and enjoy!

Bacon Pumpkin Soup

Ingredients

- ½ lb of bacon (cut to an inch size chunks)
- 2 cups of pumpkin puree
- ½ diced onion
- 2 pieces of celery stalks (diced)
- 4 slices of carrots (diced and peeled)
- 2 pieces of apples (cored, peeled and diced)
- 3 cloves of minced garlic
- ½ teaspoon of cinnamon (ground)
- ¼ teaspoon of ginger (ground)
- 1 tablespoon of olive oil
- 4 cups of chicken stock
- ¼ cup of pumpkin seeds (toasted)
- Pepper and salt for tasting

Directions

1. Cook bacon in a large sized pot until it becomes crispy. Remove and put on a plate lined with paper towels. Set aside and let cool.

2. Remove bacon fat. Using the same pot, add olive oil, carrots, celery, and onions. Sauté for about 5-7 minutes or until onions become translucent.

3. Add apples and cook for 3-5 minutes or until it begins to caramelize. Add cinnamon, ginger, garlic and continue to cook for another minute or two until it becomes fragrant.

4. Add pumpkin puree and stock. Crank the heat to high and bring to boil. Once boiled, reduce heat and simmer for about 20 minutes.

5. Transfer soup on a food processor or you can also use a hand blender. Blend until it becomes smooth. Season to taste.

6. Ladle a good of amount of soup into bowls. Top with pumpkin seeds and bacon crisps.

7. Serve hot and enjoy!

Spicy Jicama Shoestring Fries

Ingredients:

- 1 piece of large Jicama (spiralized into noodles)
- 2 tablespoons of olive oil for drizzling
- Pinch of salt to taste
- 1 tablespoon of powdered onion
- 2 tablespoons of cayenne pepper
- 2 tablespoons of powdered chili

Directions:

1. Preheat your oven to 405 degrees.

2. Place your Jicama noodles on a baking tray and cut them into small sized noodles making them look like shoestring fries.

3. Drizzle them with olive oil and lightly toss to evenly coat the noodles.

4. Season the Jicama noodles with salt, cayenne pepper, powdered onion and powdered chili. Again lightly toss them so that the spices and seasoning will be evenly distributed. Make sure not to overcrowd the noodles to avoid sticking together.

5. Bake for 15 minutes then turn it over to bake them again for another 10 to minutes or until your preferred crispiness.

6. Serve hot and enjoy your snack!

Quick Corn Salad

Ingredients:

- 1 cup frozen corn
- 1 tablespoon green pepper, chopped
- 2 green onions, sliced thinly
- ¼ cup fat-free mayonnaise
- ¾ teaspoon ground mustard
- 2 tablespoons lemon juice
- ¼ teaspoon sugar
- Salt and Pepper to taste
- Leaf lettuce *(optional for garnish)*

Directions:

1. In a small mixing bowl, combine the ground mustard, mayonnaise, lemon juice, and sugar. Mix until well blended. Stir in the corn, green pepper, and green onions. Add salt and pepper to taste. Cover and

refrigerate for about 4 hours. Serve on leaf lettuce if desired.

Easy Bake Kale Chips

Ingredients

- 1 tablespoon of olive oil or coconut oil

- 3 to 4 kale leaves

- Spice mixes such as pepper, oregano, thyme, basil, red pepper flakes and sage (depends on your preference)

Directions

1. Preheat your oven to 350 degrees F.

2. Rinse kale and shred leaf. Discard the stem.

3. Using a resealable bag or plastic container, add the olive oil, kale leaves and your preferred spices. Seal and toss the ingredients until leaves are all thoroughly coated.

4. Spread the leaves in a sheet pan. Make sure that the leaves are opened sufficiently to ensure cooking.

5. Bake the kale leaves for about 12 minutes or until it becomes crisp on its edges.

6. Remove and place on a bowl to cool for a few minutes. Enjoy!

Cucumber and Blueberry Smoothie

Ingredients

- 1 cup of coconut milk
- 1 tablespoon of lemon juice
- 2 pieces of a large cucumber (diced and peeled)
- 1 cup of blueberries (frozen)

Directions

1. Place all of the ingredients in your blender. Blend until smooth.
2. Transfer to a glass and enjoy!

Apple Baked Chips

Ingredients

- 2-3 pieces of apples
- Cinnamon (ground)

Directions

1. Preheat your oven to 220 degrees F.

2. Line your sheet pan using parchment paper then set aside.

3. Meanwhile, cut your apples into thin slices and spread them on your sheet pan. Be sure to cover them evenly and avoid overlapping. Sprinkle ground cinnamon on top and place inside the oven.

4. Bake for about hour to dry it out then flip the other side. Cook for another hour.

5. Remove from oven and let cool. Serve and enjoy!

Grain-Free Brownie Bites

Ingredients

- 1 ½ cups of walnuts
- 1 teaspoon of vanilla
- A pinch of salt
- 1/3 cup of cocoa powder (unsweetened)
- 1 cup of dates (pitted)

Directions

1. Using your food processor or blender, add salt and walnuts. Pulse until walnuts are grounded finely.

2. Add vanilla, cocoa powder and dates in the blender. Mix until well combined. While your mixer is still running, add a few amount of water just to make sure that the mixture will stick together.

3. Transfer mixture to a bowl and form them into balls using hands. Store inside a container. Make sure that it is airtight. This can last until a week. Enjoy!

Quinoa Veggie Salad

Ingredients:

- ½ cup quinoa, rinsed
- ½ cup frozen peas, thawed
- 1 shallot, minced
- 1 small carrot, shredded
- 1 cup grape tomatoes, cut in half
- 1 tablespoon fresh thyme, minced
- 1 tablespoon fresh parsley, minced
- 2 cups fresh spinach
- 1 cup water
- 1 tablespoon balsamic vinegar
- 2 tablespoons lemon juice
- 1 ½ teaspoon Dijon mustard
- 2 teaspoons olive oil

- ¼ teaspoon sugar

- 1/8 teaspoon pepper

- ¼ teaspoon salt

Directions:

1. In a small-sized saucepan, bring the water to a boil. Add the quinoa. Reduce the heat, cover and simmer for about 12 to 15 minutes or until the liquid is fully absorbed. Remove from the heat then fluff with a fork. Transfer the cooked quinoa in a large bowl and let cool completely. Add the grape tomatoes, peas, shallot, and carrot.

2. In a small mixing bowl, combine the balsamic vinegar, lemon juice, thyme, parsley, olive oil, Dijon mustard, sugar, pepper, and salt. Drizzle over quinoa mixture and toss until everything is well coated. Chill until serving. Once ready to serve, place the spinach in the serving plate then top with the quinoa salad.

Mint, Cucumber and Green Apple Smoothie

Ingredients

- Juice of half a lime
- ½ cup of Greek yogurt (non-fat)
- ¼ cup of cucumber (chopped and peeled)
- 1 small sized green apple (sliced and cored)
- ¼ cup of baby spinach (fresh)
- ½ teaspoon of mint (fresh)
- ¼ cup of coconut water (unsweetened)
- 2 cups of ice

Directions

Place all of the ingredients in your blender. Blend well until smooth. Transfer to a glass and enjoy!

Kale and Pear Smoothie

Ingredients

- ½ cup of peeled green grapes
- ½ of pear (chopped)
- ½ of peeled orange
- ½ cup of kale
- A cup of water
- 1 piece of banana (chopped)
- 2 cubes of ice

Directions

Place water, orange, kale and grapes in your blender. Blend over slow speed for about 60 seconds then add banana, pear and the ice cubes. Blend until smooth. Transfer to a glass and enjoy!

FINAL WORDS

Thank you again for purchasing this book!

I really hope this book is able to help you.

The next step is for you to **join our email newsletter** to receive updates on any upcoming new book releases or promotions. You can sign-up for free and as a bonus, you will also receive our "*7 Fitness Mistakes You Don't Know You're Making*" book! This bonus book breaks down many of the most common fitness mistakes and will demystify many of the complexities and science of getting into shape. Having all this fitness knowledge and science organized into an actionable step-by-step book will help you get started in the right direction in your fitness journey! To join our free email newsletter and grab your free book, please visit the link and signup: **www.hmwpublishing.com/gift**

Finally, if you enjoyed this book, then I would like to ask you for a favor, would you be kind enough to leave a review for this book? It would be greatly appreciated!

Thank you and good luck in your journey!

ABOUT THE CO-AUTHOR

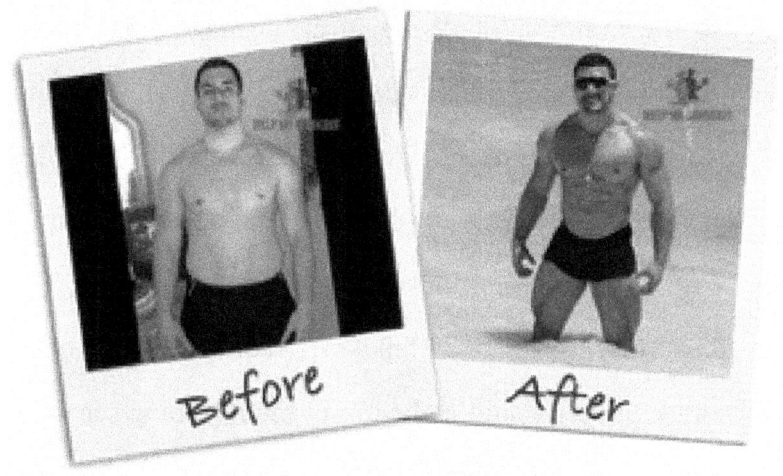

My name is George Kaplo; I'm a certified personal trainer from Montreal, Canada. I'll start off by saying I'm not the biggest guy you will ever meet and this has never really been my goal. In fact, I started working out to overcome my biggest insecurity when I was younger, which was my self-confidence. This was due to my height measuring only 5 foot 5 inches (168cm), it pushed me down to attempt anything I ever wanted to achieve in life. You may be going through some challenges right now, or you may simply want to get fit, and I can certainly relate.

For me personally, I was always kind of interested in the health & fitness world and wanted to gain some muscle due to the numerous bullying in my teenage years about my height and my overweight body. I figured I couldn't do anything about my height, but I sure can do something about how my body looked like. This was the beginning of my transformation journey. I had no idea where to start, but I just got started. I felt worried and afraid at times that other people would make fun of me for doing the exercises the wrong way. I always wished I had a friend that was next to me who was knowledgeable enough to help me get started and "show me the ropes."

After a lot of work, studying and countless trial and errors. Some people began to notice how I was getting more fit and how I was starting to form a keen interest in the topic. This led many friends and new faces to come to me and ask me for fitness advice. At first, it seemed odd when people asked me to help them get in shape. But what kept me going is when they started to see changes in their own body and told me it's the first time that they saw real results!

From there, more people kept coming to me, and it made me realize after so much reading and studying in this field that it did help me but it also allowed me to help others. I'm now a fully certified personal trainer and have trained numerous clients to date who have achieved amazing results.

Today, my brother Alex Kaplo (also a Certified Personal Trainer) and I own & operate this publishing venture, where we bring passionate and expert authors to write about health and fitness topics. We also run an online fitness website "HelpMeWorkout.com" and I would love to connect with by inviting you to visit the website on the following page and signing up to our e-mail newsletter (you will even get a free book). Last but not least, if you are in the position I was once in and you want some guidance, don't hesitate and ask... I'll be there to help you out!

Your friend and coach,

George Kaplo
Certified Personal Trainer

Get another book for Free

I want to thank you for purchasing this book and offer you another book (just as long and valuable as this book), "Health & Fitness Mistakes You Don't Know You're Making", completely free.

Visit the link below to signup and receive it:

www.hmwpublishing.com/gift

In this book, I will break down the most common health & fitness mistakes, you are probably committing right now, and I will reveal how you can easily get in the best shape of your life!

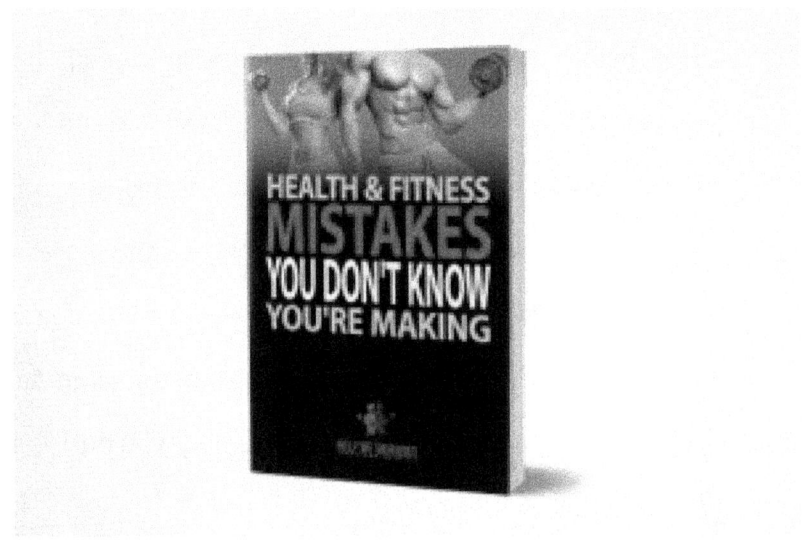

In addition to this valuable gift, you will also have an opportunity to get our new books for free, enter giveaways, and receive other valuable emails from me. Again, visit the link to sign up:

www.hmwpublishing.com/gift

Copyright 2017 by HMW Publishing - All Rights Reserved.

This document by HMW Publishing owned by the A&G Direct Inc company, is geared towards providing exact and reliable information in regards to the topic and issue covered. The publication is sold with the idea that the publisher is not required to render accounting, officially permitted, or otherwise, qualified services. If advice is necessary, legal or professional, a practiced individual in the profession should be ordered.

From a Declaration of Principles which was accepted and approved equally by a Committee of the American Bar Association and a Committee of Publishers and Associations.

In no way is it legal to reproduce, duplicate, or transmit any part of this document in either electronic means or in printed format. Recording of this publication is strictly prohibited, and any storage of this document is not allowed unless with written permission from the publisher. All rights reserved.

The information provided herein is stated to be truthful and consistent, in that any liability, in terms of inattention or otherwise, by any usage or abuse of any policies, processes, or directions contained within is the solitary and utter responsibility of the recipient reader. Under no circumstances will any legal responsibility or blame be held against the publisher for any reparation, damages, or monetary loss due to the information herein, either directly or indirectly.

The information herein is offered for informational purposes solely, and is universal as so. The presentation of the information is without contract or any type of guarantee assurance.

The trademarks that are used are without any consent, and the publication of the trademark is without permission or backing by the trademark owner. All trademarks and brands within this book are for clarifying purposes only and are the owned by the owners themselves, not affiliated with this document.

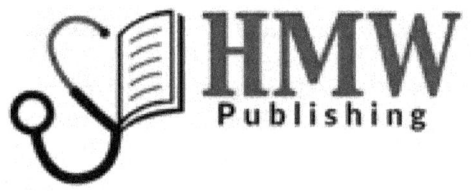

For more great books visit:

HMWPublishing.com

www.ingramcontent.com/pod-product-compliance
Lightning Source LLC
Chambersburg PA
CBHW071113030426
42336CB00013BA/2060